# PAWSITIVELY

## GEORGIA - BE BRAVE, IMPRESS YOURSELF, BE YOUR OWN BREED

ELIZABETH FERRIS

This book is dedicated to you.

Positively Georgia — Be Brave,
Impress Yourself, Be Your Own Breed



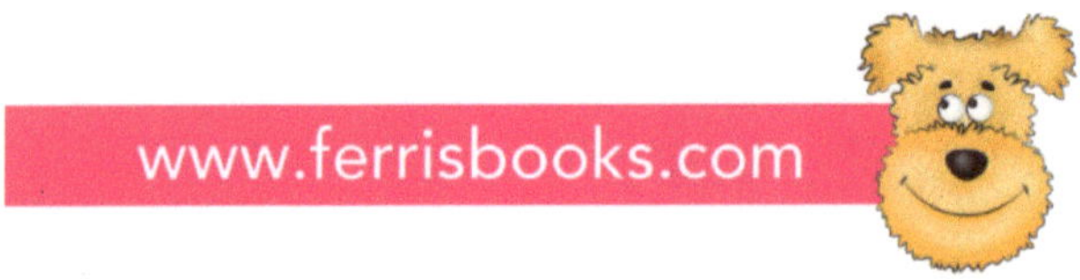


Illustrations: Matrix Solutions
Editor: Neil Shooter
Layout: Sumbal Tariq

ISBN
978-1-7779086-1-4 (Hardcover)
978-1-7779086-0-7(Paperback)
978-1-7779086-2-1(eBook)

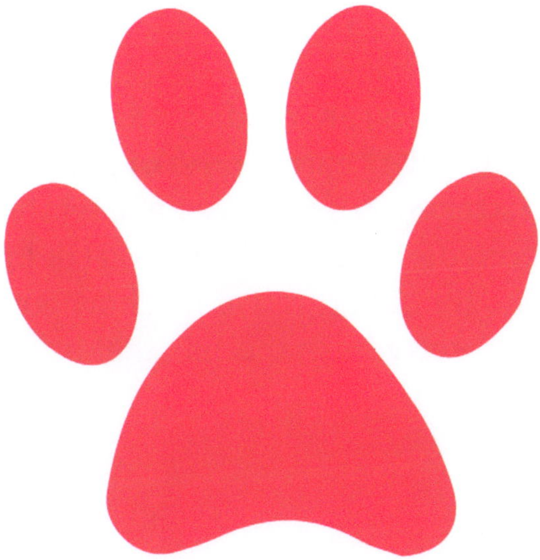

The year is 2021. If you are reading this book in the future, you may have heard stories of people wearing masks and partaking in excessive hand washing. This is true. I was born during a Pandemic and I didn't know any better and thought this was just how humans lived. They did smell pretty fresh though, that is for sure.

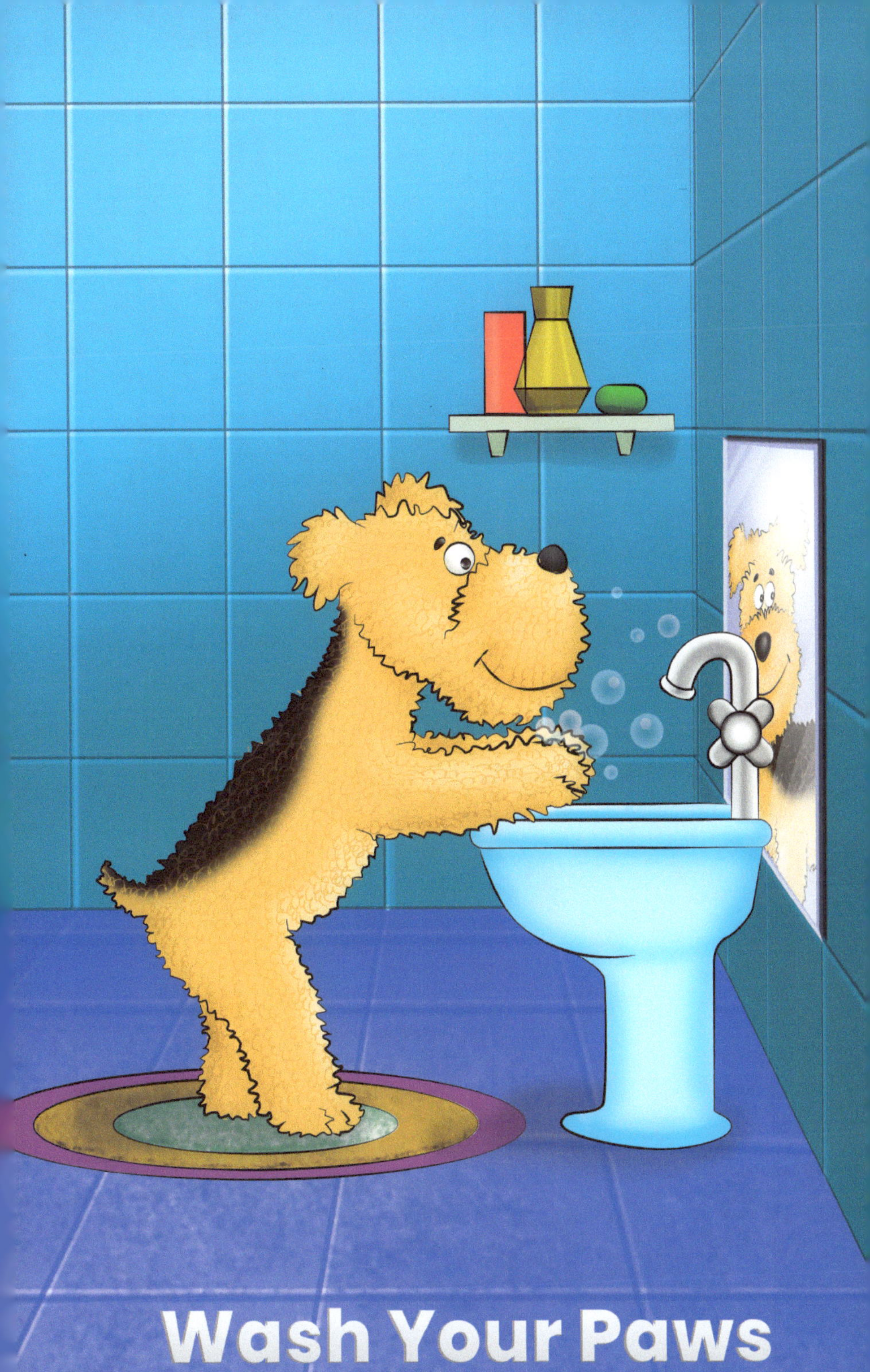

# Wash Your Paws

My name is Positively Georgia. My owner, Norman, calls me "Georgie-girl" for short and I am an Airedale Terrier puppy with a very positive outlook on life. I live in Northwestern Canada. I am a motivational, furry soul. I'm having such a great time on this planet being a unique therapy dog. I help people realize their natural abilities, and inspire them to achieve all those things they want to have, do, and become.

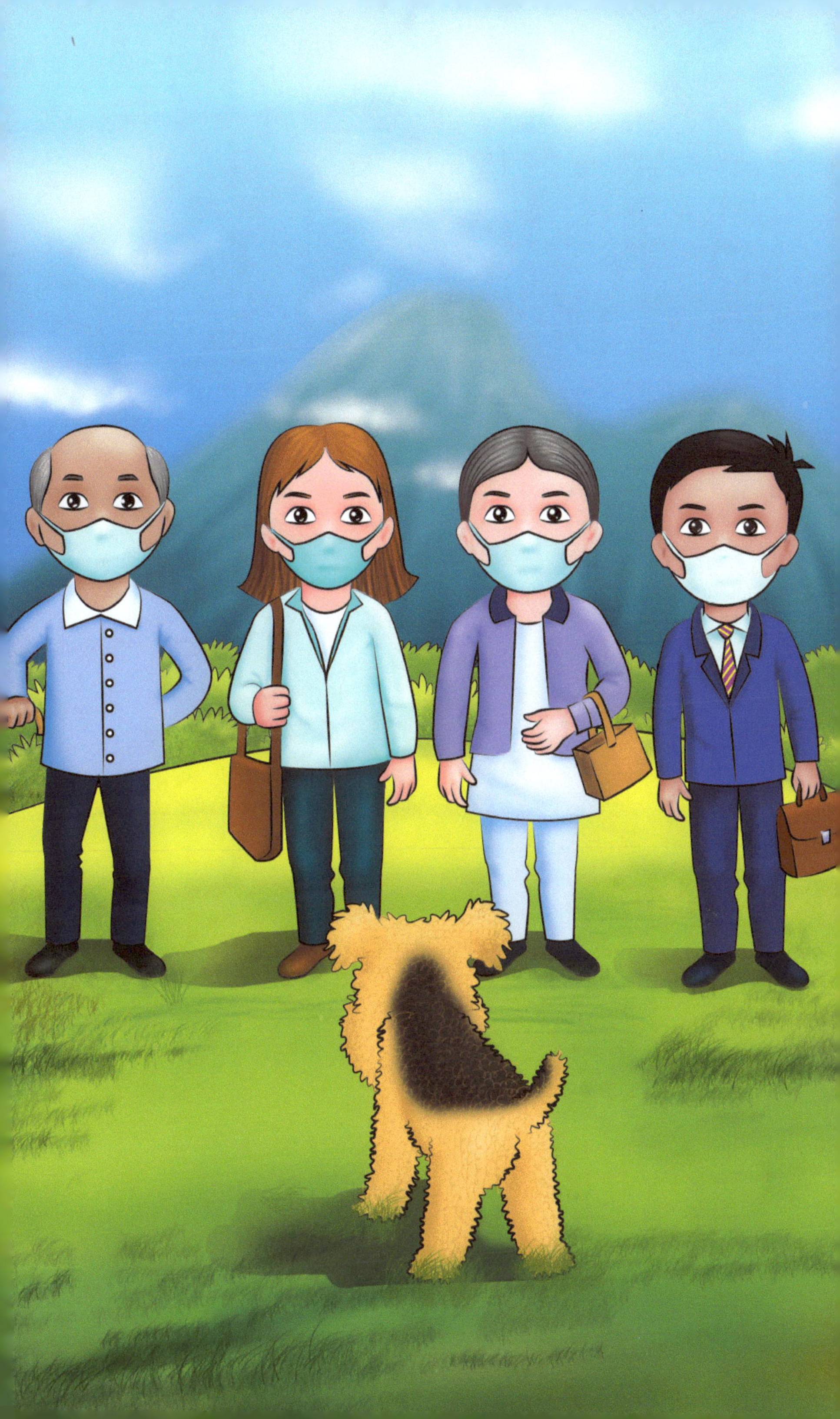

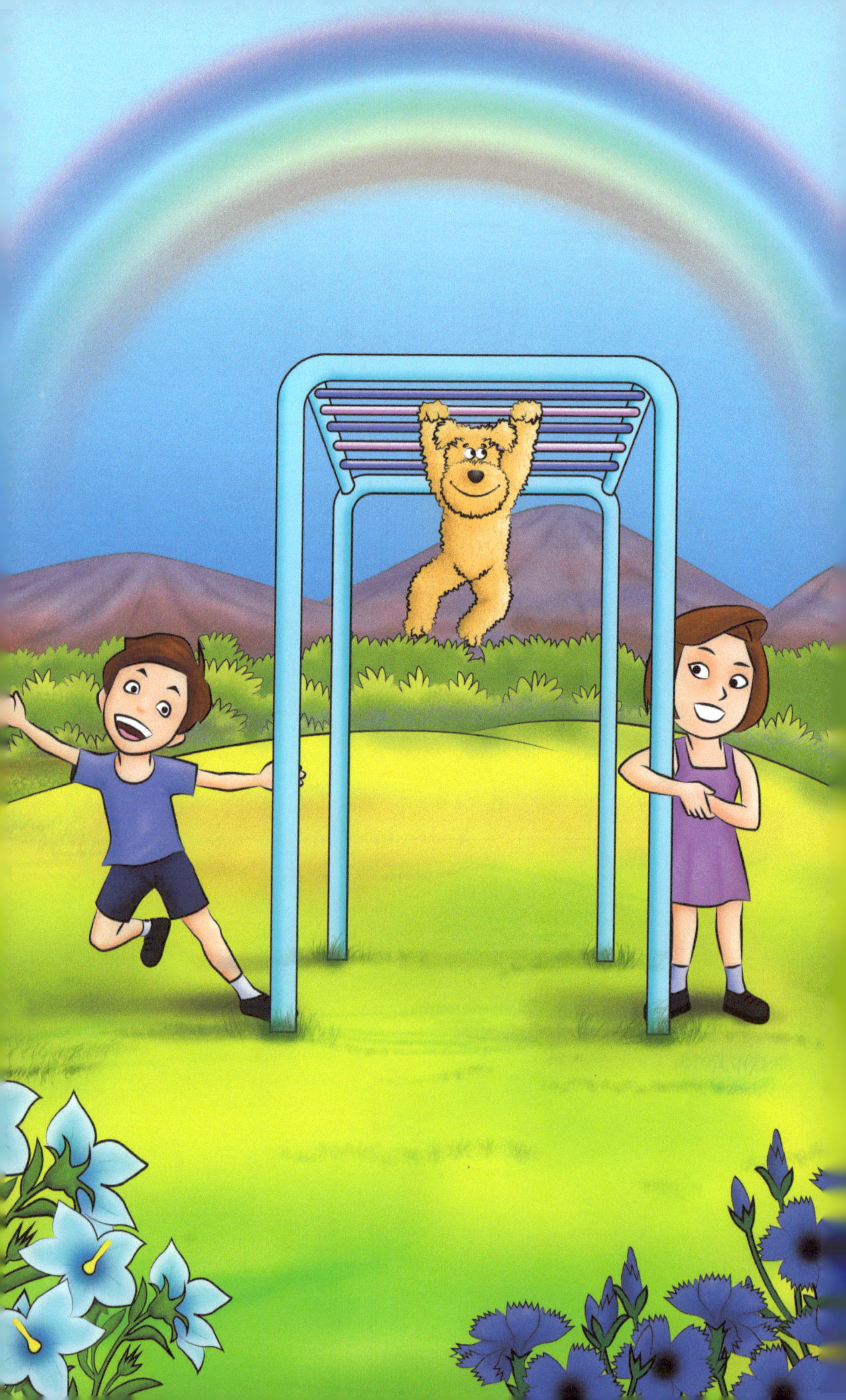

I have such big goals and dreams of how I might be a benefit to the world, and really want to help others succeed by barking out my thoughts for all to hear. I love turning my dreams into reality, and I hope my thoughts inspire you to do this also, my dear readers. That is why I decided to create this book on being brave and how to truly impress yourself. I want you to feel so good about yourself inside and out, like I do, that you wish you had started barking sooner. Woof!

When you live through a Pandemic, like I did, you really begin to appreciate every moment even more. You have to be brave and keep the faith within you alive. It was a crazy time, but I figured out how to find peace, which ultimately led to pure, unwavering happiness within my furry soul that beamed out, and I knew I just had to share this with the world.

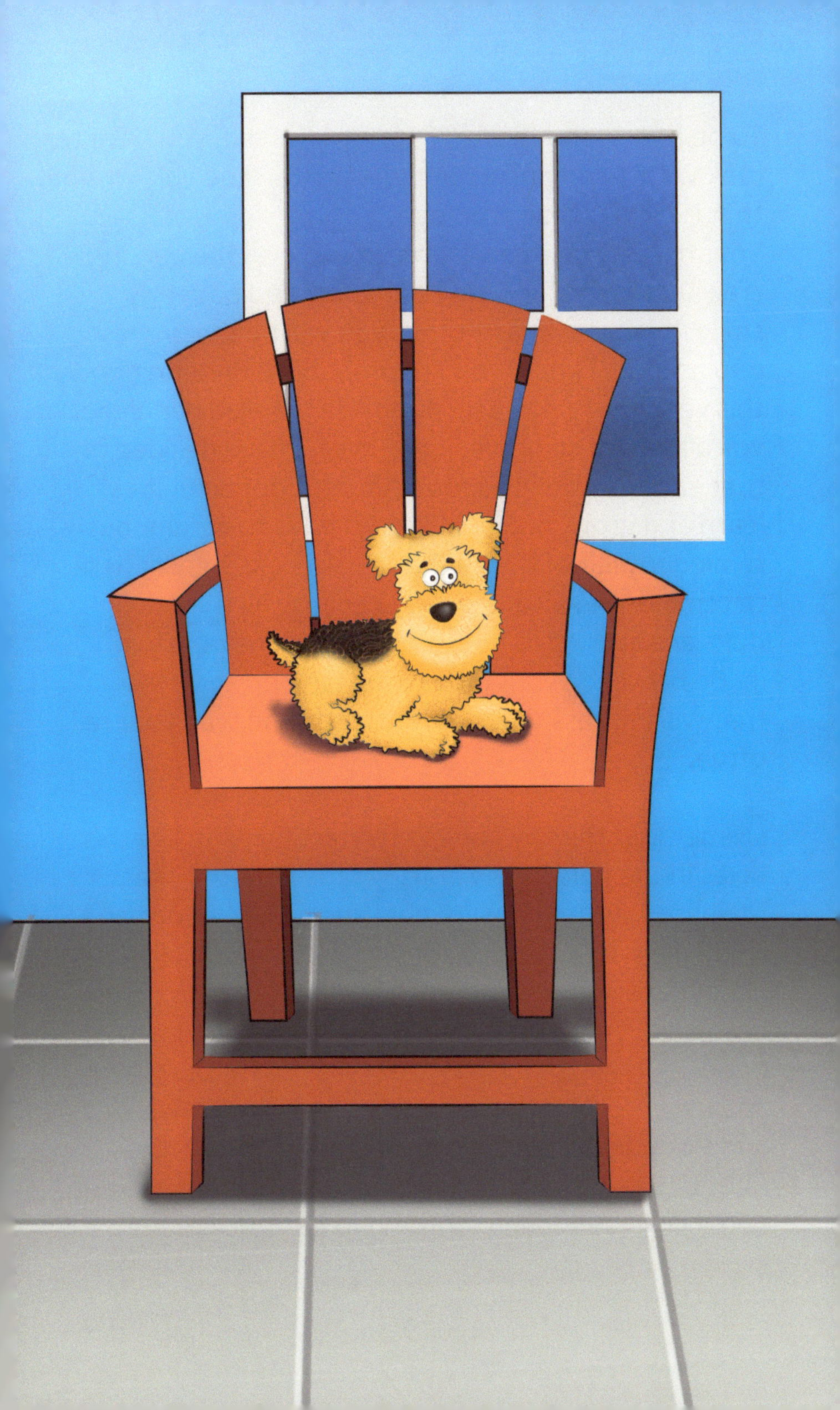

To be brave, and to truly impress yourself, you have to look within and find your higher self — the voice inside that is calmer than your ego.
Your higher voice can calmly observe all the barking craziness of life, and stay centered, and patiently smile. If you can master this, you will be the bravest pup around. I know you are probably wondering how this very young Airedale puppy discovered her higher voice and got so brave, right? Well, I have decided that each day brings about different opportunities to learn and grow, but I will admit I have to continuously remind myself of the direction I am heading. I'm here to remind you, also, that just because all the other dogs are barking, it doesn't mean you have to join in. Be brave, be your own breed, and do something that will impress yourself. Be happy and wag your tail often.

I remember the day I began to start thinking like this. I was in the field by my house in the country. That is where I live with my owner, Norman. My Norman is the best. He takes me for walks in the sunshine almost every morning, which is great because then I can enjoy many different spots to have big, giant poops. Anyways, one day we were out for our walk, and I was sniffing the tasty bits of hay and flowers, and I wandered a little farther than I normally do, right to the very end of my long leash and slipped out of my collar. Suddenly, these two gigantic creatures appeared from the long grass. They scared me so much because they were about seven times my size, or maybe even bigger! Huge, gigantic creatures with massive wings that opened up with a very loud WHOOSH!

Right away, my Norman called out to me, "Georgie-girl! Come here!"

I ran as fast as I could. The two gigantic creatures took flight and I felt this huge, dark cloud of shadows looming over my furry head. I felt shivers in every nerve of my body. My heart was pounding and a rush of energy came over me. My furry soul screamed to my brain, "Run! Fast! Run away!"

They let out a sound so loud, so very loud, it was like a trumpet!

"Georgie-girl!" my Norman called again. "Look up! Trumpeter swans!"

At that moment, I realized the emotion I felt was definitely fear, and definitely because of those very loud noises that echoed over and over again. What in the world was a trumpeter swan? I stopped, looked up, and … wow! There they were, slowly soaring up into the blue sky. Beautiful, magnificent, gigantic birds with a massive wingspan, blasting their noises up into

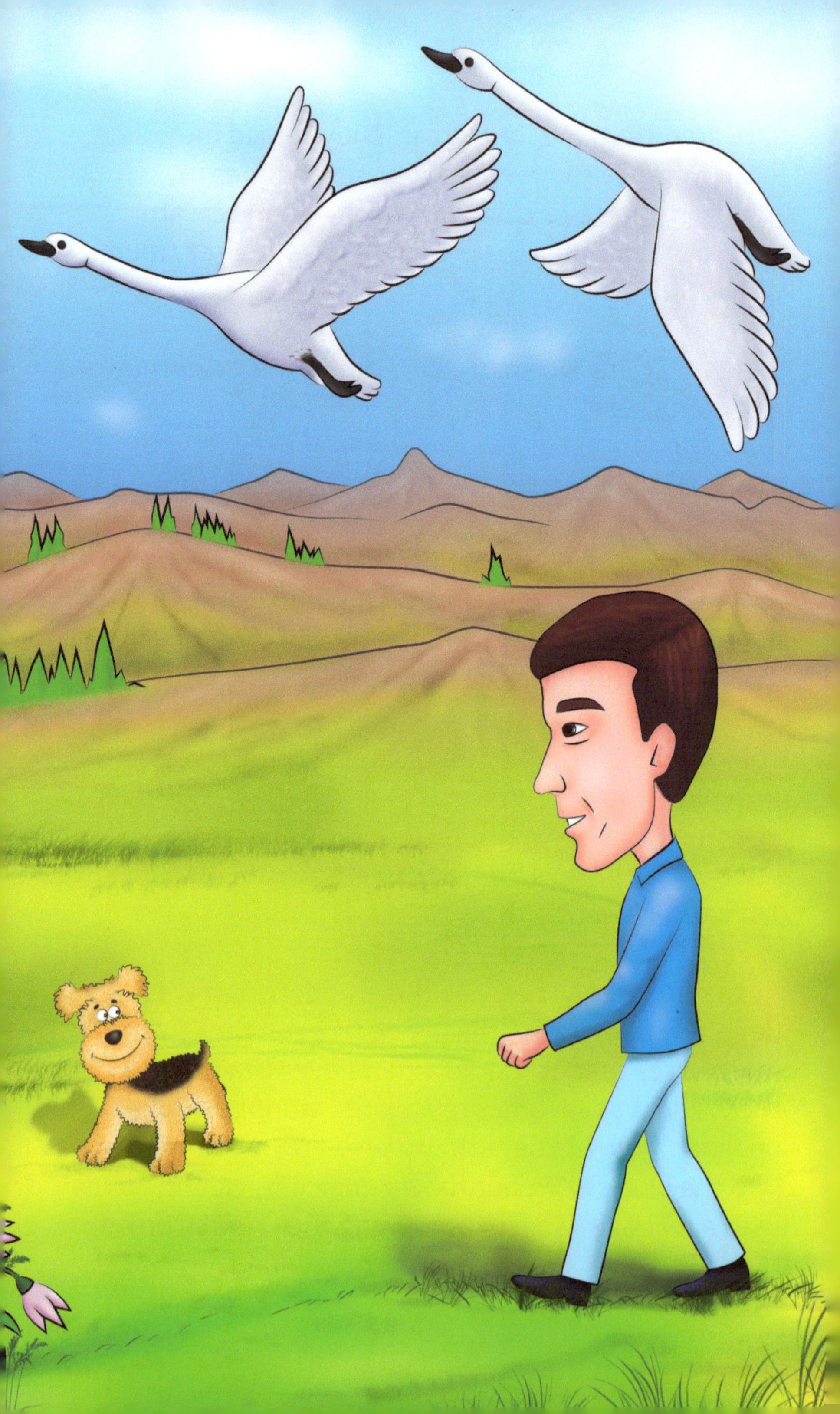

the air with such enthusiasm! As they flew off into the distance, I could still hear their calls. I realized this was the first time I had ever felt a tremendous sense of fear. It was a strange feeling, and I didn't like it. Why did the loud noises make me feel fear? I shook my furry body, determined to learn more and share what I learned with everyone who needed to hear it, so we could all be our best brave selves, and so I would never let fear take over my happy-go-lucky feeling again.

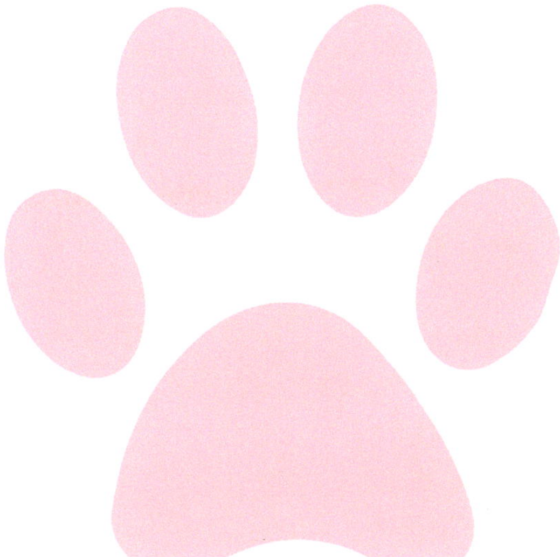

After our long walk, my Norman and I came back home, and he told me to go play while he made lunch. I let out a woof! I like play time and I like lunch! (I especially like bacon snacks, but that story is for another time. Which reminds me of a joke: What is a dog's favorite food? Anything that is on your plate! Ha! But I digress.) Sometimes, during playtime, my imagination takes me away on all kinds of travels within my mind. Later, I would learn that these were actually opportunities to discover and realize the potential of my higher self, all contained in my amazing Airedale mind. Do you make time to sit still and dream? You should, you are wonderful, and I encourage you to learn more about yourself and what is inside you waiting to be shared with the world. As I sat in the living room that wonderful day, I arranged my favourite toys around me and my imagination began to look within my own thoughts. I asked my ladybug toy, "Why was I fearful of the noise of those beautiful trumpeter swans this morning?"

My ladybug toy looked at me and whispered, "Maybe you didn't recognize the situation so your thoughts turned inward, and that caused your body to describe what happened as fearful?"

Teddy groaned, and said, "Dude … that's deep! Rather than being fearful, next time just stop … take a breath … and don't get your stuffing all up in a bunch!" Teddy laughed.

I turned to Teddy, and said, "Why do you keep calling

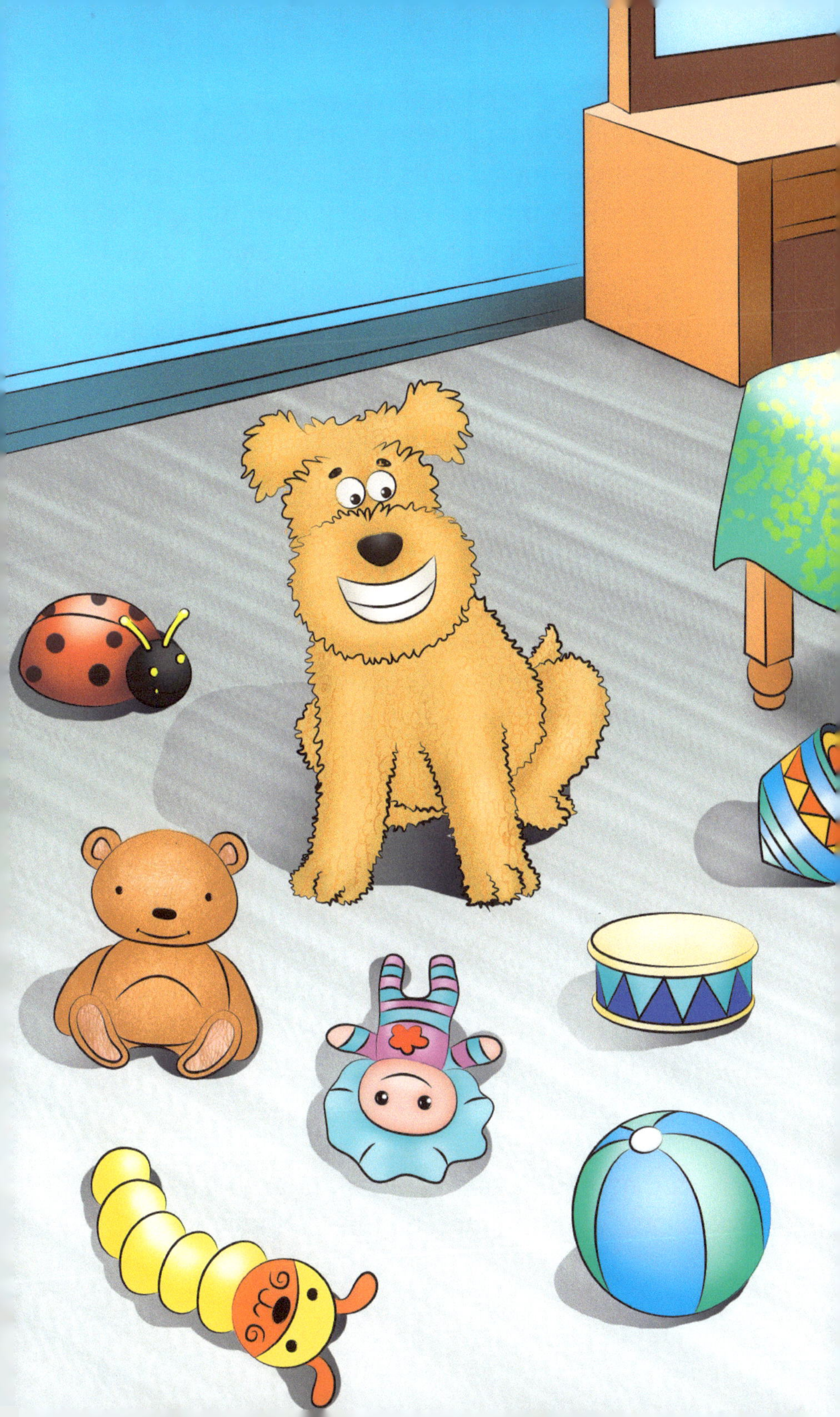

me 'dude'?" I picked up Teddy with my slobbery mouth and licked and chewed at its face. As I slurped away on its soft, sticky fur, my mind began shifting. What if I changed that feeling of fear … to a feeling of such gratitude for being able to experience that moment? I focused on the positive moment of those beautiful sources of energy flying up and away, that I was very fortunate to witness. I felt my fur starting to fluff up. I let out a big woof as I realized I was the one in control of how I feel. Being grateful for these special moments in my day makes me happy.

"Woof! Woof!"

At that moment, I also understood that if I were to let fear take over my thoughts it would make me feel sick, and this would take my mind down a path I definitely didn't want to travel down again. I thought about my Norman. I realized that instead of being fearful of the trumpeter swans, Norman has courage. I decided that next time I didn't know what something was, rather than being fearful, I would remind myself that I have the courage within, just like my Norman. Let's all be brave and impress ourselves!
Just then, I heard my Norman call out to me, "Lunch is ready, Georgie-Girl."

I dropped my teddy, and he let out a groan, and said, "Dude, careful of the merchandise!" and I ran across the wooden floor with a clickety-click, in a tap-dancing delight, getting to the kitchen as fast as I could. Teddy groaned again, and said, “Dude, why do you always leave me in a pile of your slobber? Not cool, dude. Not cool.”

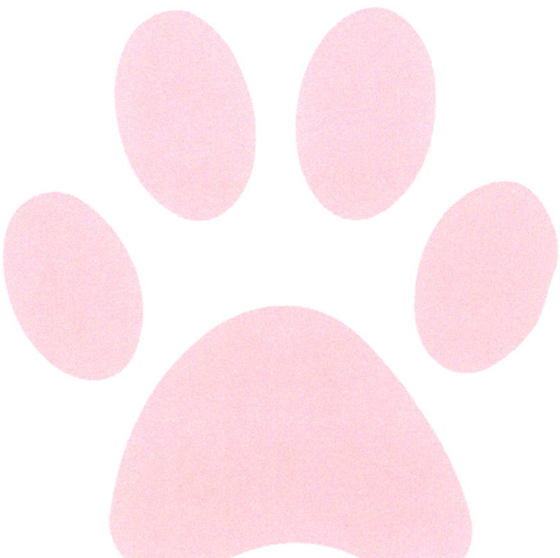

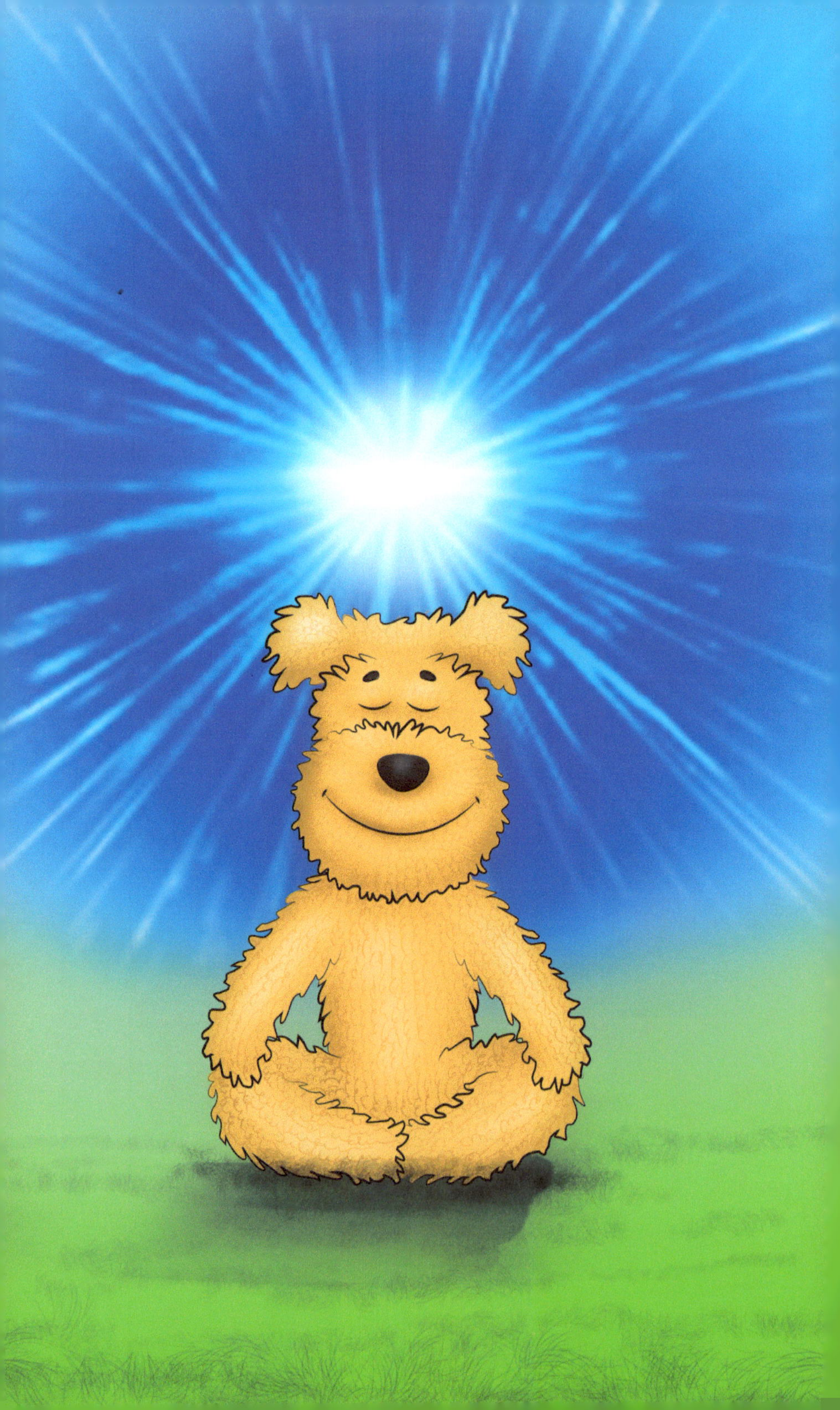

As I ate lunch my mind wandered off again, but this time into a meditative state of gratitude. It occurred to me that if all creatures had this ability to find their inner bravery and impress themselves, what a gift we would give to ourselves, and to others. I made a commitment to myself that I would always be true to myself and release all my powerful thoughts in the hopes of sharing my greater purpose to benefit others. And then I thought of another joke I heard: What do you call a large dog that meditates? Aware wolf. Ha! Yes, I know, I'm a pretty funny dog. Another one of my talents. Laughter is the key to a great life.

Do you express gratitude daily for all your dog treats, toys, experiences and the beautiful furry family and friends in your life? I do. Gratitude helps me stay focused on the positive, no matter what is happening in the world around me, even during a Pandemic.

When I concentrate on what's good in my Norman and I's life, it becomes so much easier for me to find daily creativeness, and deep joy, and I definitely feel this strength to create the kind of life I want to live. I feel like a very brave puppy for sharing this with you, and my hope is that you feel the energy within, like me, and use your gifts to do things that will impress yourself. Remember to breathe. Hope you find your inner puppy breath and share that with the world, like me. My breath smells like rawhide and bacon bits. You?

Speaking of puppy breath, can you smell it from over there? Yes, that's right. I like to dig up the occasional sunflower plant from the neighbor's yard and bring it to my Norman so he knows how much I love him and like him. One day was extra special, though, as I had the good fortune of a lucky intervention when a ladybug landed on my fur. It was a cute little ladybug with many spots. She crawled all over my furry face and then down my snout to the end of the sunflower I had in my mouth. Her name was Isabella. Isabella was sent to this Earth to bring good fortune and prosperity to everything she lands on, and everyone. She also said I would be granted one wish and it would come true. So, I promptly made a wish for more wishes to come true. That seemed like a no brainer! Ha! One of my wishes is that I will always be a dreamer. Sometimes I dream I'm by the ocean lying in a hammock and listening to the waves. One day, while I was dreaming, I heard the neighbors talking, and they said their dog ate florescence crayons and was pooping out what looked like Easter eggs all over the lawn.

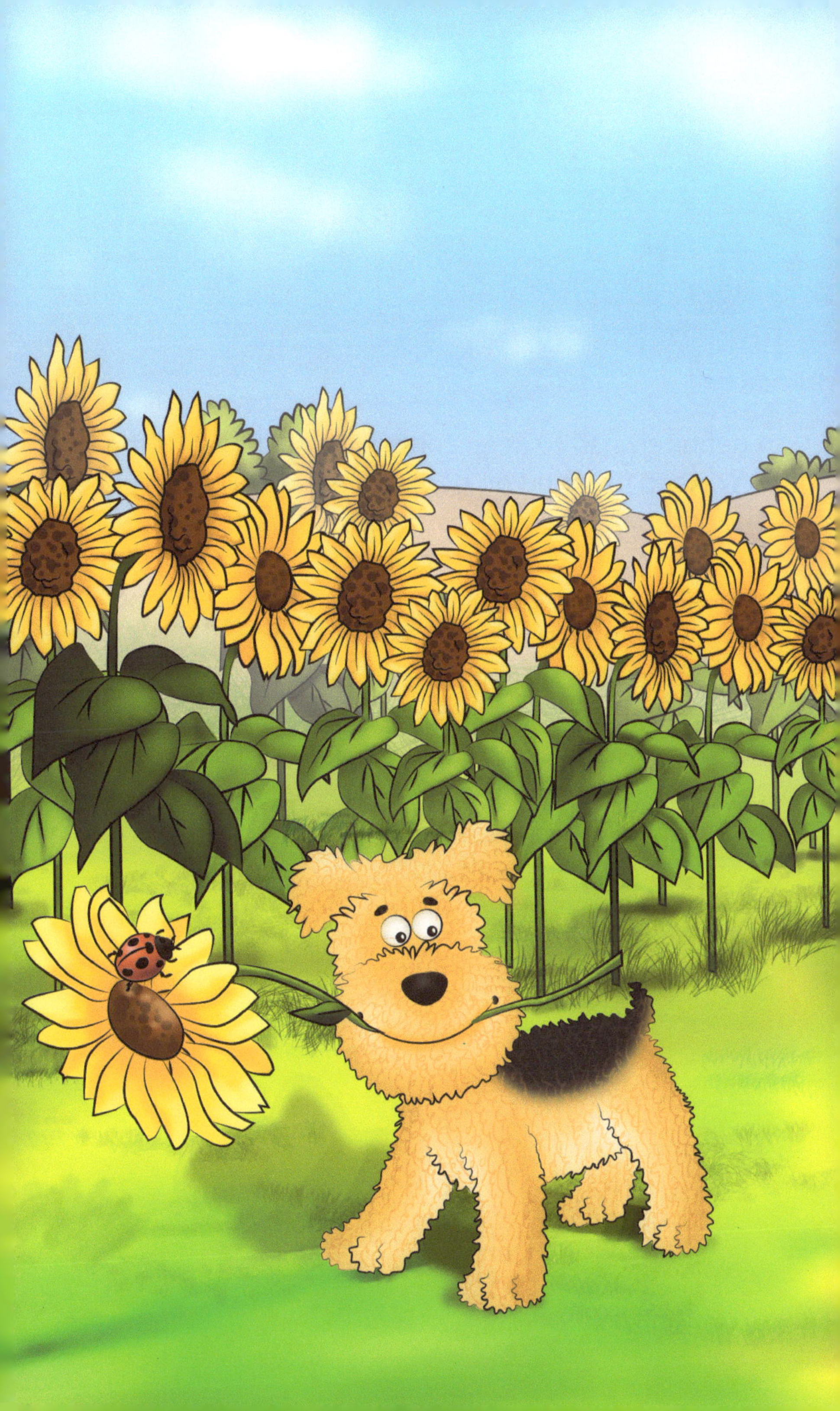

I definitely had to keep control of my thoughts that day, keep my mind on track, not go down the rabbit hole of thoughts, and resist the urge to go look. I like being capable of imagining, and then taking that thought and bringing it into form. I feel so very proud of myself for realizing this. It's like being an instant superhero. I believe that if you can control your thoughts, then you will control your life. I've often heard my Norman say, "Anything you believe, you can achieve. It all starts in your mind!" Do you ever get the chance to be a superhero? I hope so. It is so very "woof!" to like yourself.

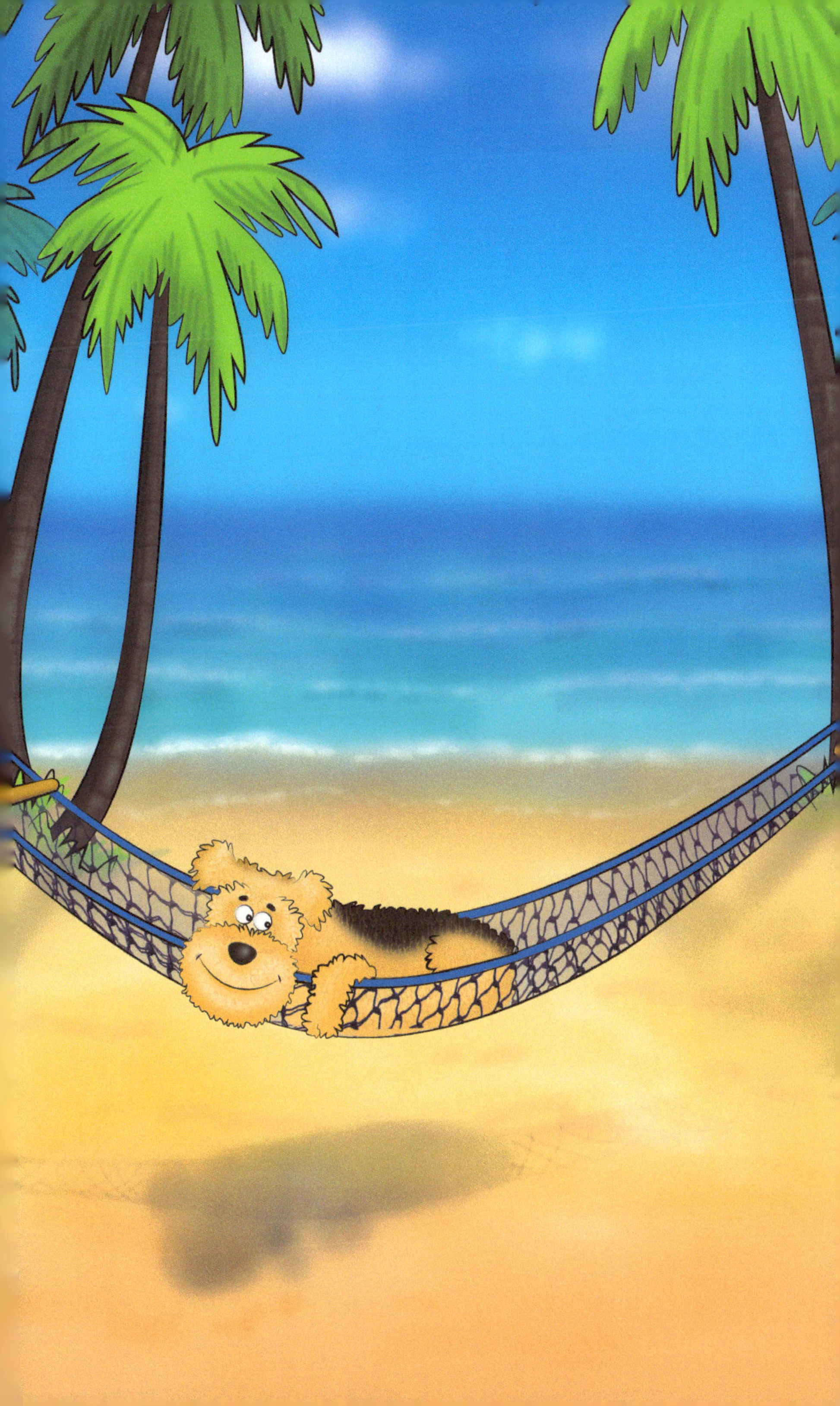

One day, I even had a superhero cape. OK, it was a "cone of shame" because I had to go to the veterinarian and get an operation, and it was put on to stop me from chewing at my fur. I like to joke and say that I can hear sounds 55 miles away, and my Norman got better cell phone reception that day. But I digress. Ha!

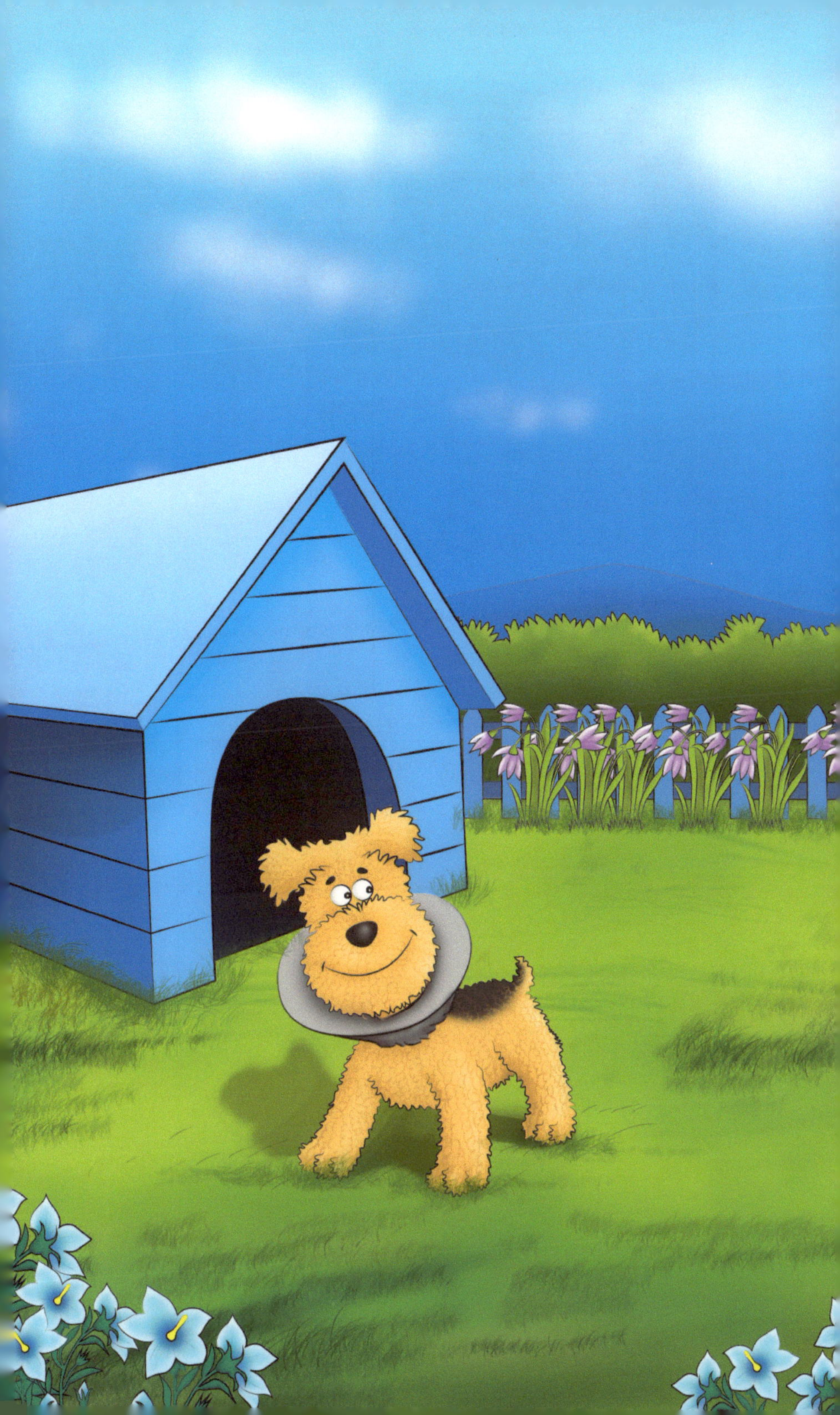

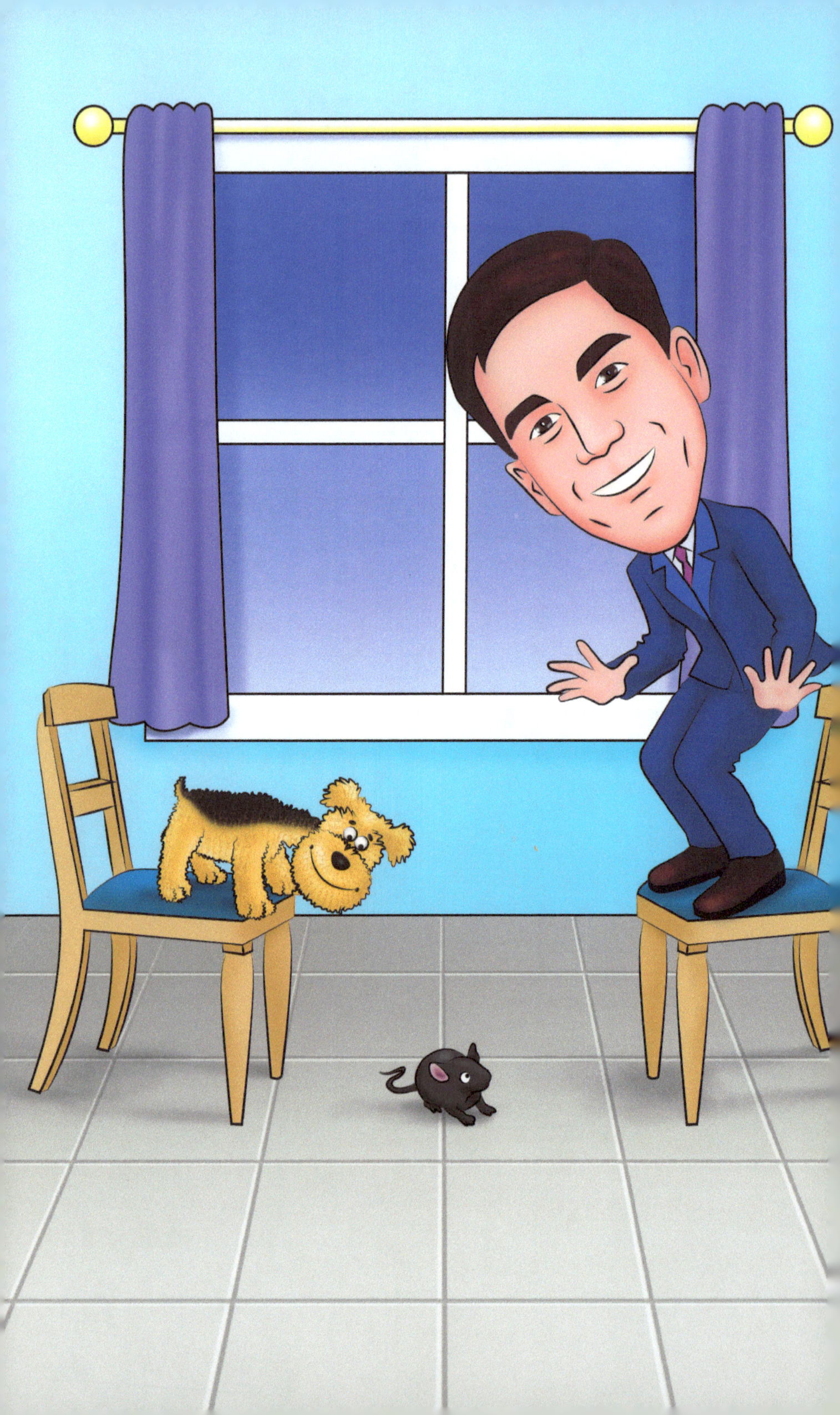

My Norman is really such an inspiration to me and those who get to cross his path. He is so kind and really is one of my favorite humans in the entire world. He is so silly too. One day a mouse ran across our kitchen floor. My Norman jumped up on a chair, which in turn caused my furry self to also jump up onto a chair.

The mouse looked at us both and said, "Scared of me?"

My Norman said, "Nope!" with a big smile. "I'm just playing musical chairs."

Have you heard of musical chairs, dear reader? Well, I've recently learned that this game involves setting up chairs with one fewer chair than the number of creatures. While music plays, the participants walk around the set of chairs. When the music stops, all players must quickly find their own individual chair. The player who fails to sit on a chair is eliminated. A chair is then removed for the next round, and the process repeats until only one player remains and is declared the winner. It's a silly game, and I've often wondered what the prize is at the end — I mean, do you get to keep the bunch of chairs? Ha! Anyways, back to my Norman and the mouse.

"Everyone is scared of me," the mouse said. "Why are you not afraid?"

My Norman said, "You are just in the wrong place at

the wrong time. We are all connected through energy, and your energy just travelled through our house, when really you were trying to get outside to your house. You didn't mean to make us afraid of you. You were just being you." My Norman then jumped off the chair and went over to open the back door, and the mouse quickly ran out as fast as he had appeared. I could tell by my Norman's smile that he was impressed with himself for figuring this all out. I learned that day that fear is sometimes a natural part of life but it doesn't have to control one's thoughts. You can redirect your imagination and visualize positive outcomes. Be brave! Impress yourself!

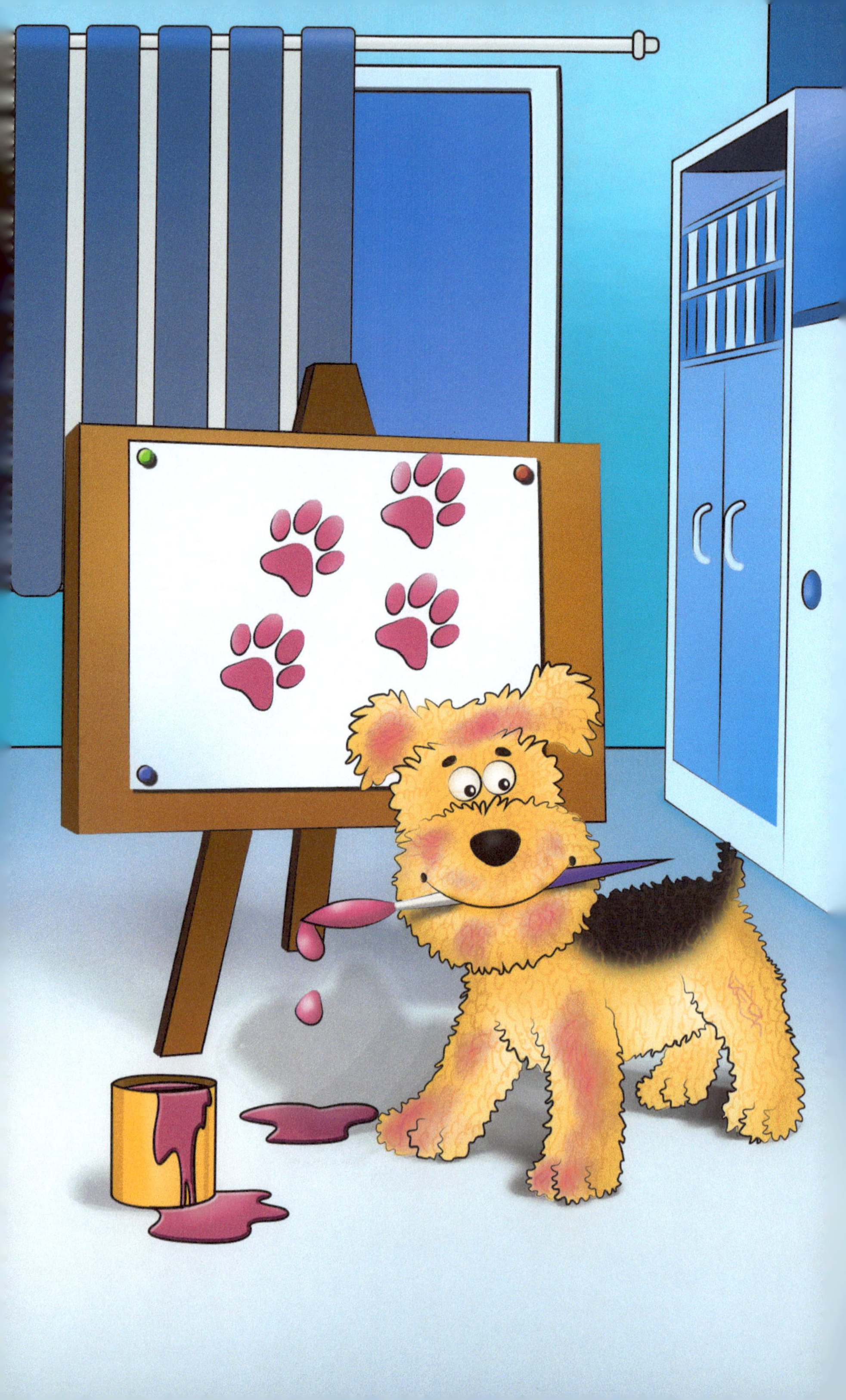

And if you want to be silly, I guess play a game of musical chairs, or paint with your paws, like I do! I will say though, dear reader, that sometimes fear is necessary to keep you safe, but do not spend time expecting a thing you do not want. I think if you spend time thinking of what you don't want, it will eventually show up, because the mind is a magnet.

I've been on several walks in the bushes in the country, and I see humans who have put bells on their dogs to keep the bears away. My Norman calls them "dinner bells". Ha! I've only thought about running into a bear once. I decided that, if this happens, I will back away slowly and never dwell on it again. It takes bravery to keep your fears from taking over your thoughts or controlling your actions. Every time I am able to not let fear or worry control my behavior, I feel impressed with myself for guiding my thoughts and learning to focus in on my puppy emotions in a way that is healthy, not harmful. I hope by sharing my puppy thoughts with you, this will help you focus on what is important as well: you, being your best self. To help with staying focused and really continuing to hold onto my braveness, I like to hang out with other creatures who are only the best and brightest, and who are always encouraging me and making me laugh. It really helps to stay away from creatures with the personality of a "wet blanket". Ha!

I like to learn from people who allow me to learn and grow, and I don't waste any time or energy on creatures who are on a mission to bring everyone around them down.

Speaking of unique creatures, once in a while I sneak over to the deluxe cat house down the road. There is a little cat door and I like to surprise my two new

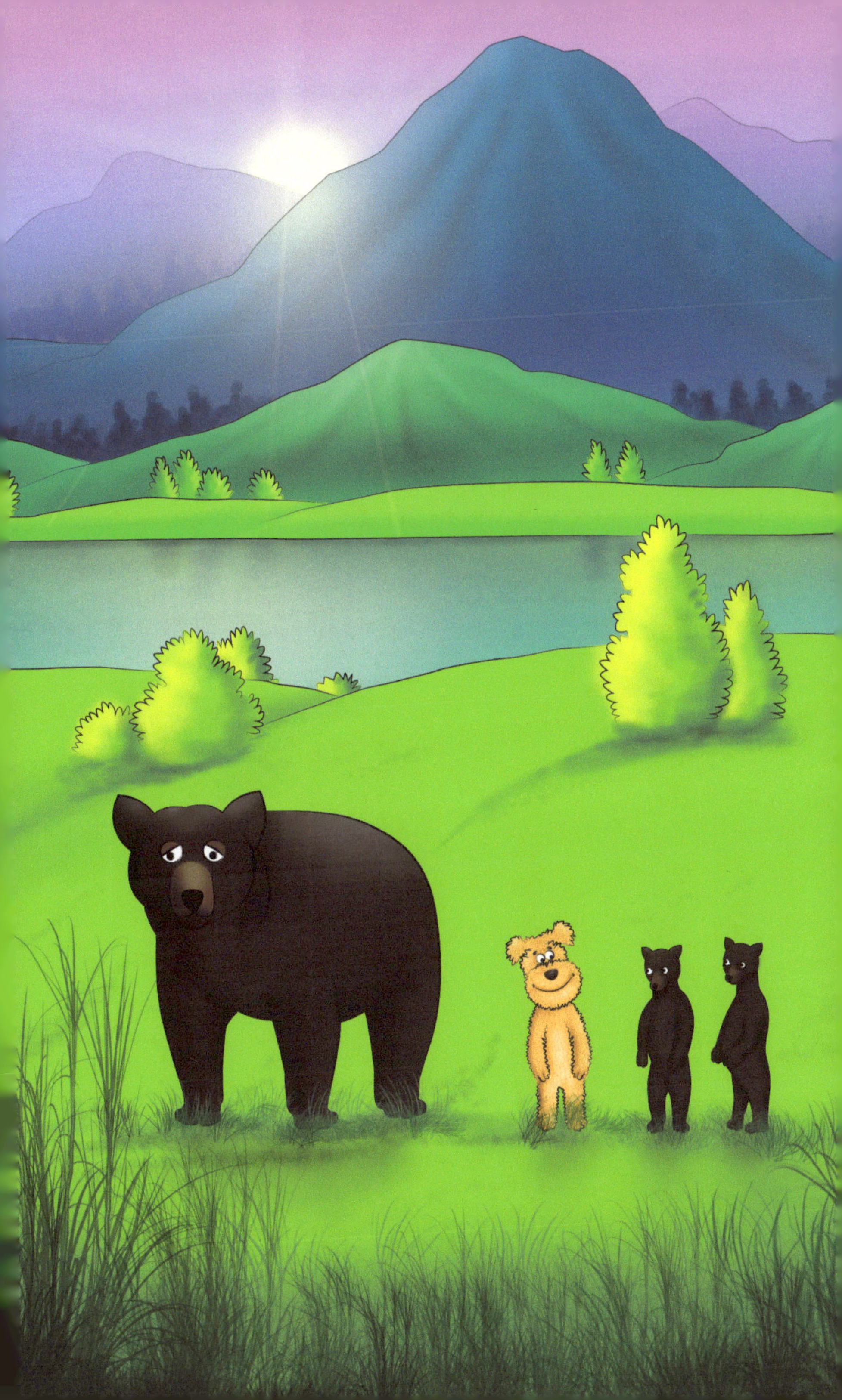

friends, Boo and Jinxer. Boo is a Ragdoll and Jinxer is a Maine Coon.
They are huge cats and, when they stretch out, they are bigger than me! Last time I was visiting them, I told them that I would be letting the world know about them, and they both said, “We want a contract, stylist, and a cage of live mice!” Ha!

They are pretty funny cats, but equally smart. Jinxer likes to sit on top of the highest perch in the house and give mini meow lectures to Boo, on the art of obsessing on goals and never giving up. Jinxer and Boo are pretty impressed with themselves and I think that is a great quality to have, as you can see the confidence beam out of their shiny eyes.

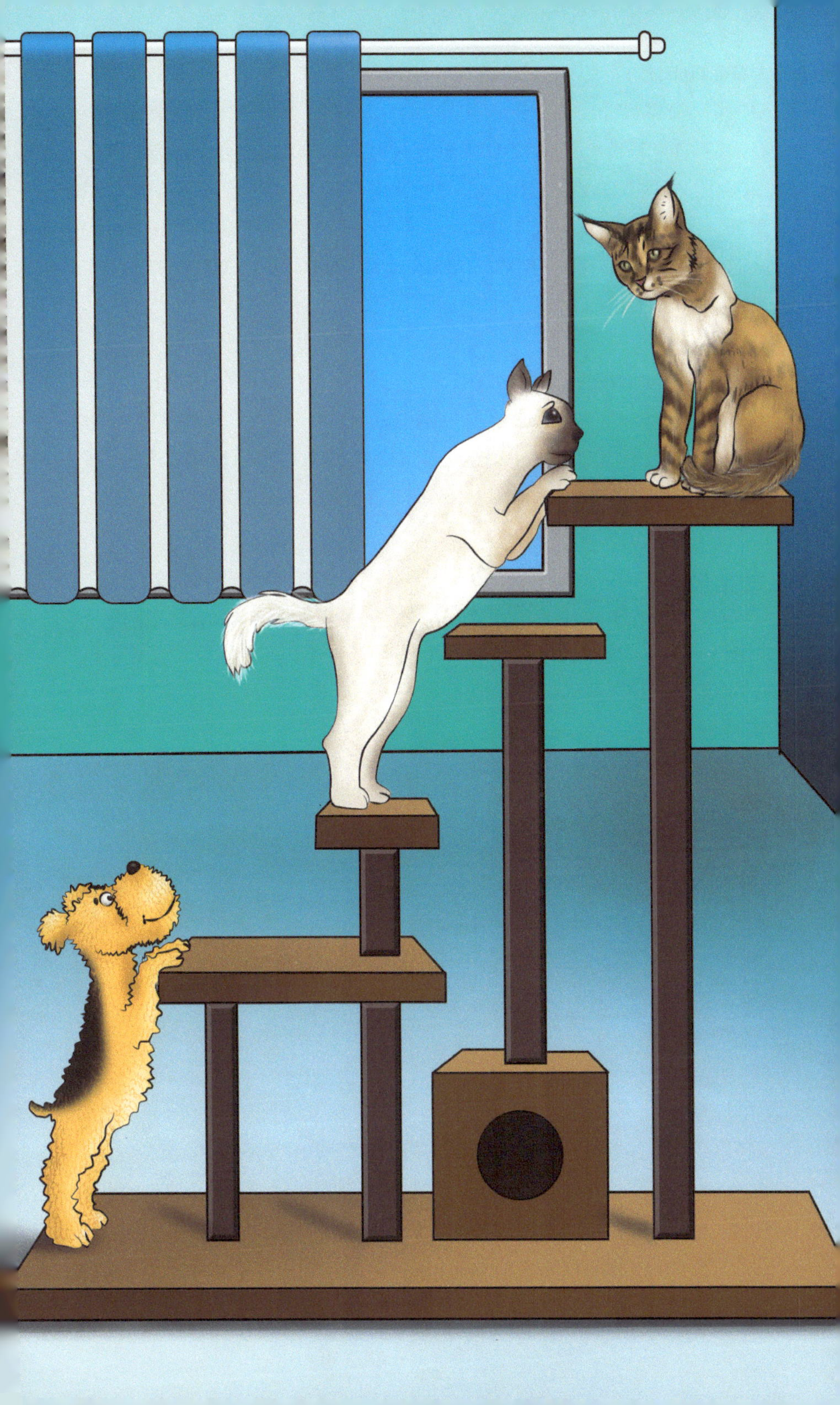

Boo doesn't give lectures like Jinxer, but quietly meows to me, "Never let anyone convince you to quit on your goal or dream. When someone tries to bring you down, remember to meow, and know that they are not really talking to you — they are meowing about their past selves that didn't follow through, and quit, and failed."

Jinxer is super-obsessed about being successful. In fact, she is. She has trained her owner to take her for walks outside on a leash, and wait for hours until she has tormented all the mice in and around the forest.

Boo is so successful that she has also trained her owner to chauffer her around to other cities to ensure she receives the latest and greatest stuffed toy, and the highest quality catnip.

These two cats really have learned how to take control over their lives — and still have all nine! There's a fun fact I learned from Boo and Jinxer. In ancient Egypt, cats were sacred animals that were worshiped as gods. Ancient Egyptians believed that cats were divine creatures with psychic or supernatural powers, and that they had multiple lives.

Boo and Jinxer definitely have superpowers as they planted this seed in my head to be in this book and — POOF! — here they are! They set goals and their goals come true! They also taught me how to meow. I think that's a pretty neat trick for a puppy to do! They also said I can come over and use their pool anytime I want!

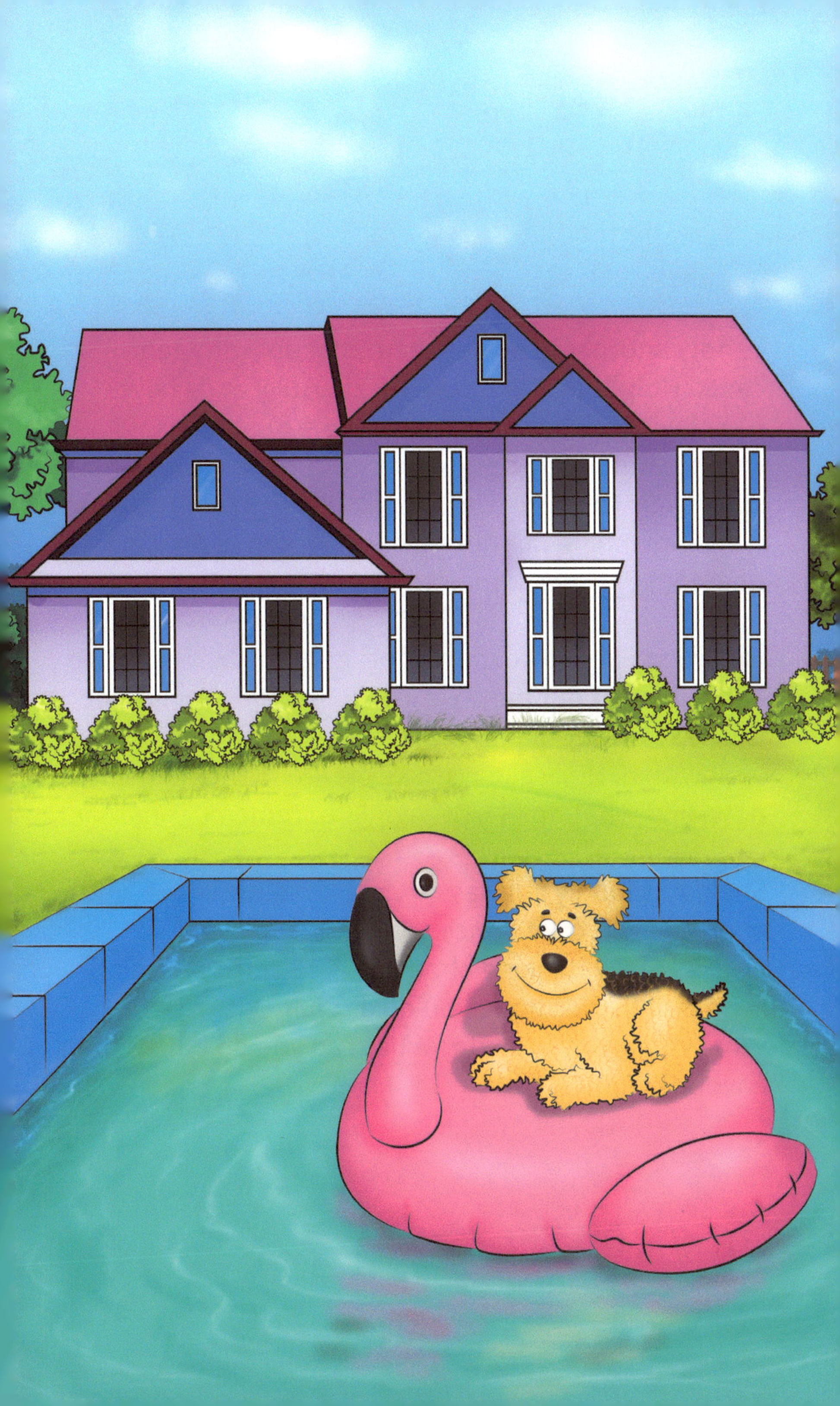

I know another level-headed furry soul with goals, called Holly. She is a Bison-Shitzu. Holly and I have fun playing in the snow. We had the best time last Christmas building a snowman together. We became so efficient in rolling the snow balls with our noses that we are planning our next creation — an entire snow dog house village complete with dog sculptures.

Holly and I like to keep each other going by reminding each other of our purpose in this life. We figured out the best way to find our purpose is to really think and look within. Holly always asks me what excites me right now, and what do I want people to remember me for.

She barks loudly and says, "Dream big, be brave, and impress everyone — including yourself!" I get so excited really thinking about what I want. I've found my passion and I hope you do as well, dear readers. What do you want to do? What can you do better than anyone else?

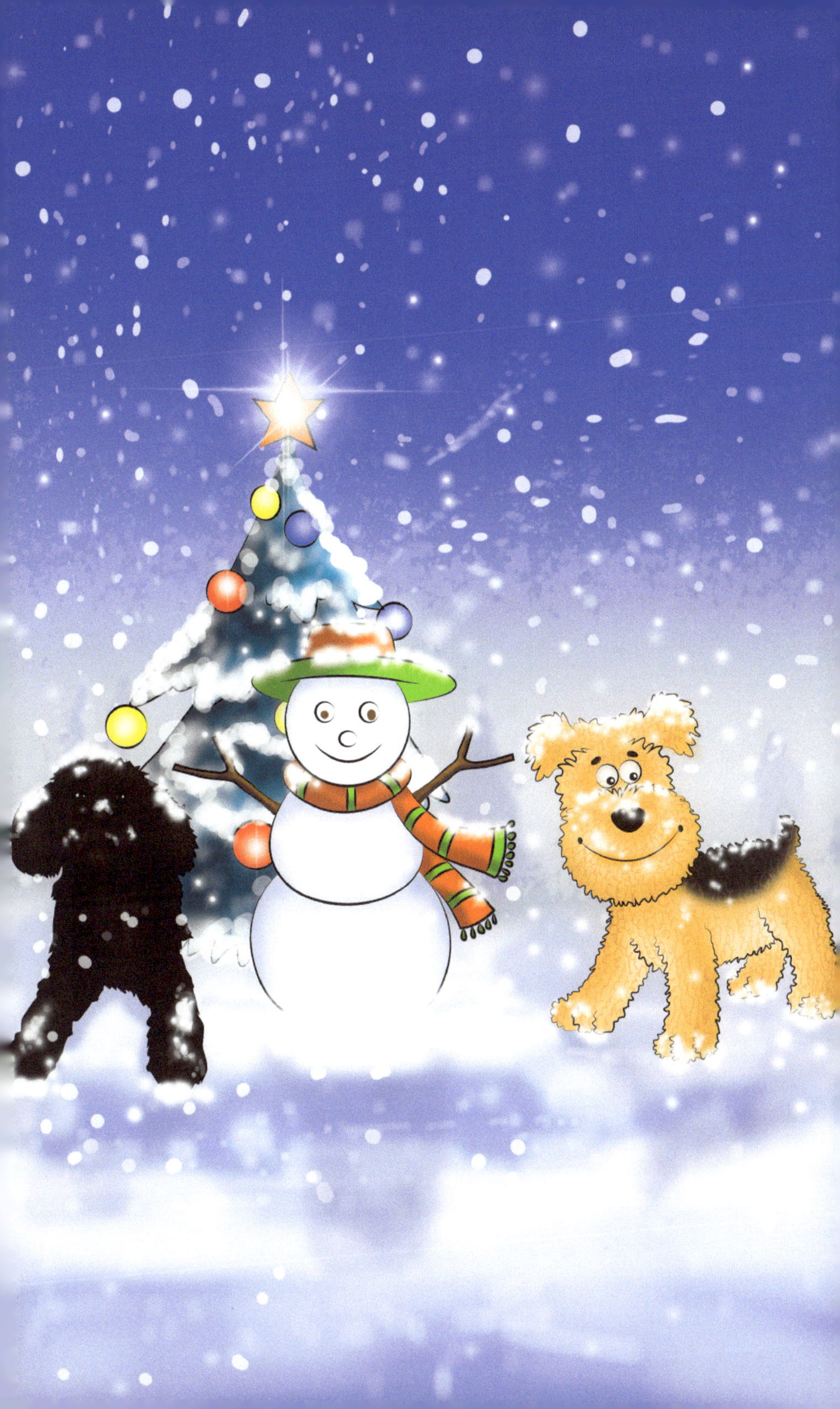

Some nights my Norman and I like to gaze up into the sky and dream big thoughts. My Norman says that it is one thing to dream but you also have to take action and follow through on your dreams, otherwise they are just wishes. My Norman is very successful because he has allowed himself to be passionate with achieving his goals

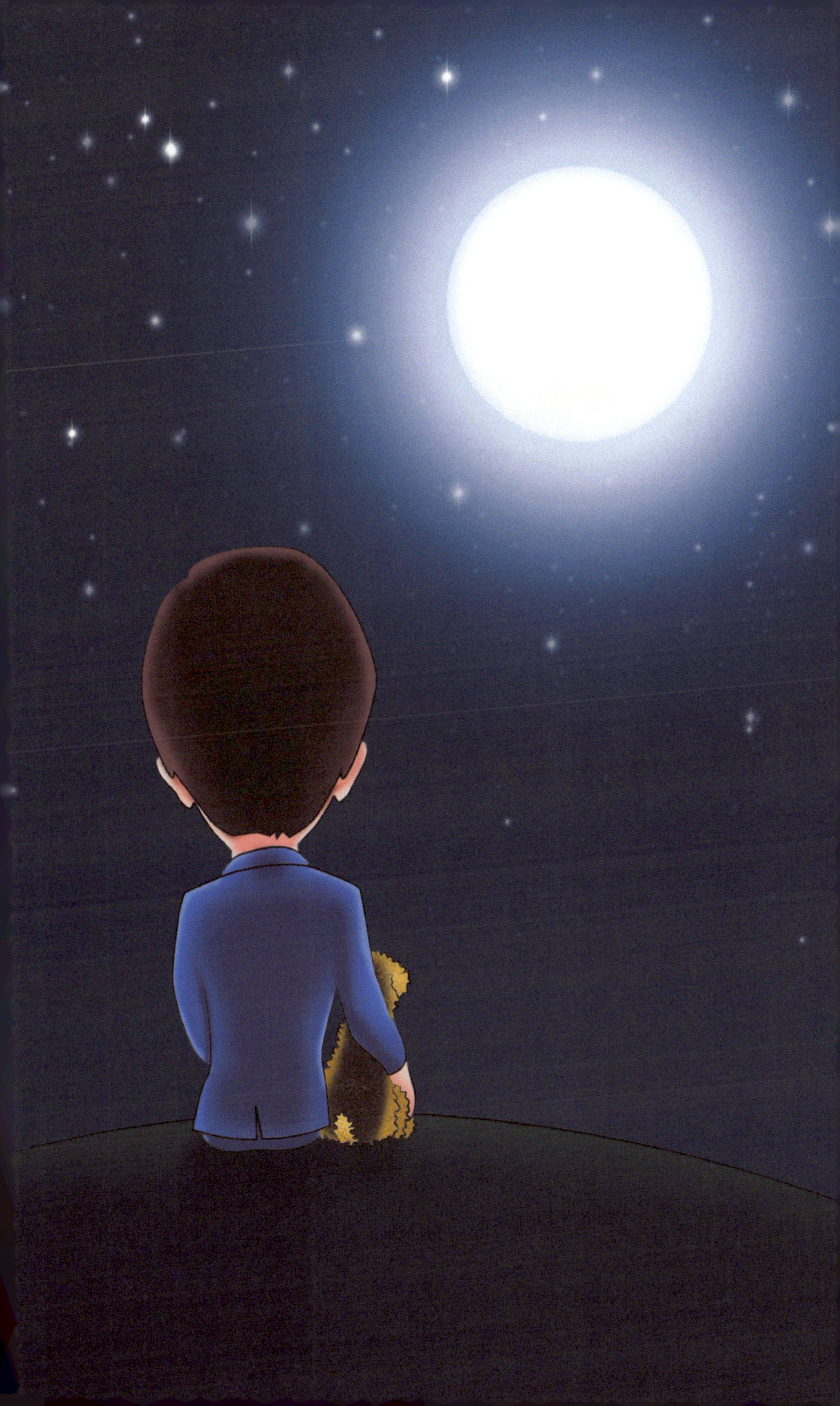

Find your passion, dear readers. The world needs you in it, and looks forward to seeing what you can create! Be brave! Impress yourself! Express your uniqueness! Your body is an extraordinary conductor of power.
I like being a unique therapy dog. I used my thoughts to create this book in the hopes of changing the world one reader at a time. Woof!

Speaking of changing the world, let me tell you even more about my Norman. By day (and sometimes into the night) he is a very successful realtor.

Sometimes he gives such inspiring talks to groups and individuals that I feel very lucky to be a little sponge soaking up his words.

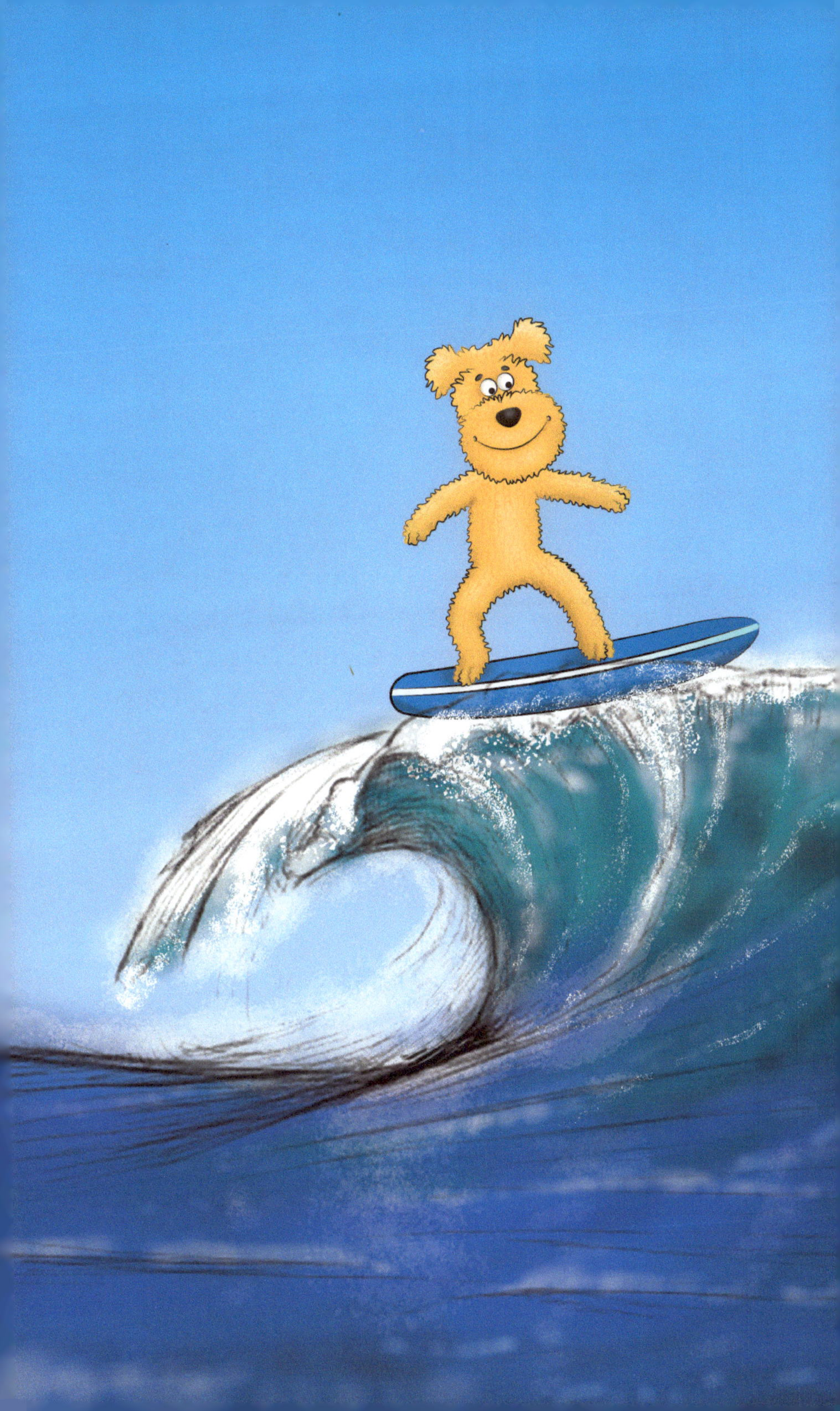

He says things like, "Wherever you are, be there." He says, "If you enjoy your here and now, and consciously experience everything you feel, think, say and do — you can really grow." How cool is that? We all have such a powerful mind that is just waiting for us to use it to its full extent.

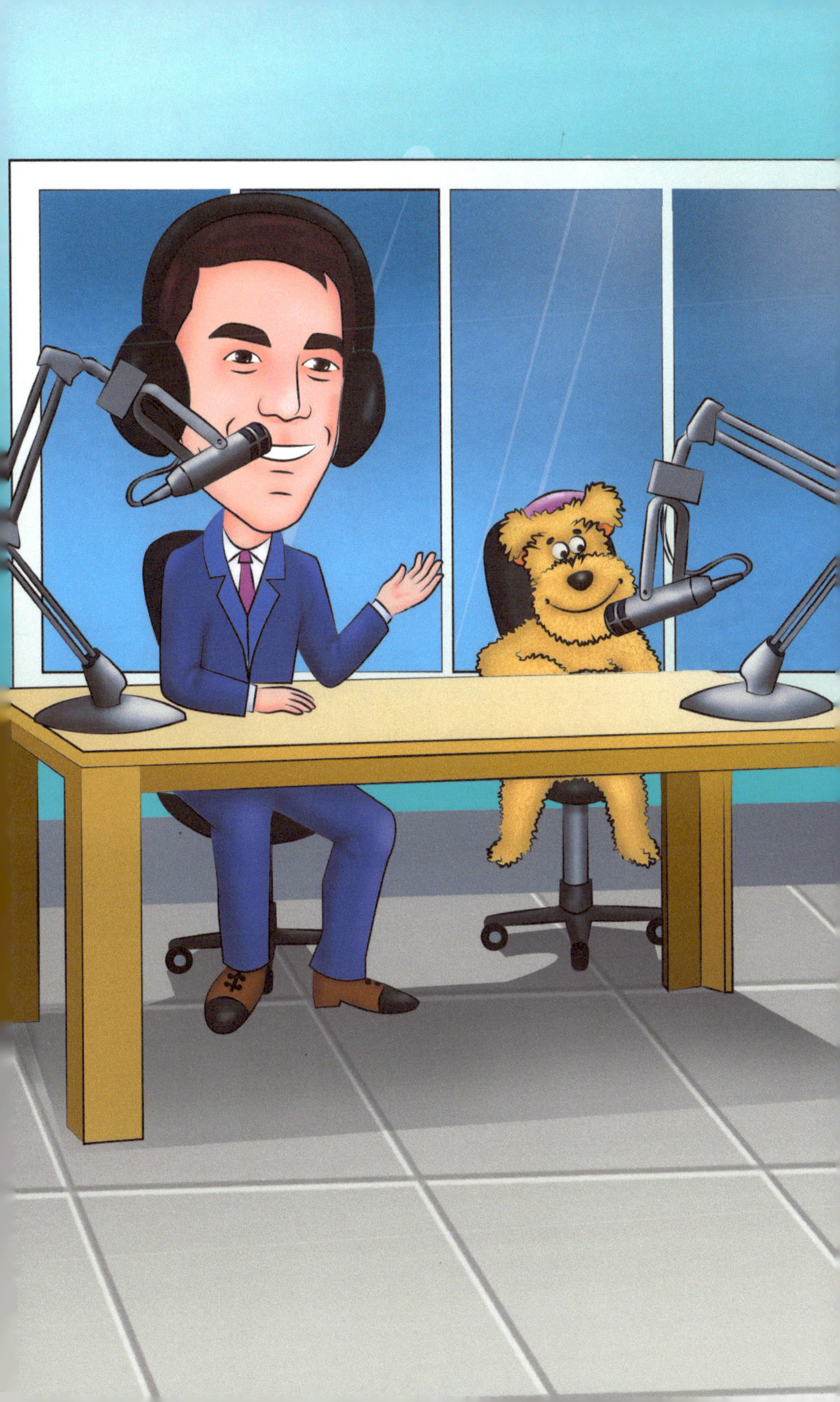

When my Norman has to go somewhere without me, sometimes I spend my day daydreaming out the living room window even more.

I see squirrels, bunnies, and birds, and even the occasional deer. It's a beautiful spot to rest and really express thanks for the wonderful things around me. Do you say "Thank You", dear reader, for the wonderfully beautiful things around you? I think it's really important to be appreciative of this world we live in. I think life is miraculous.

I think you are perfect, you have always been perfect, and you will always be perfect. The essential you. Every day that you get to be brave and express the real, genuine you, you should be impressed with yourself!

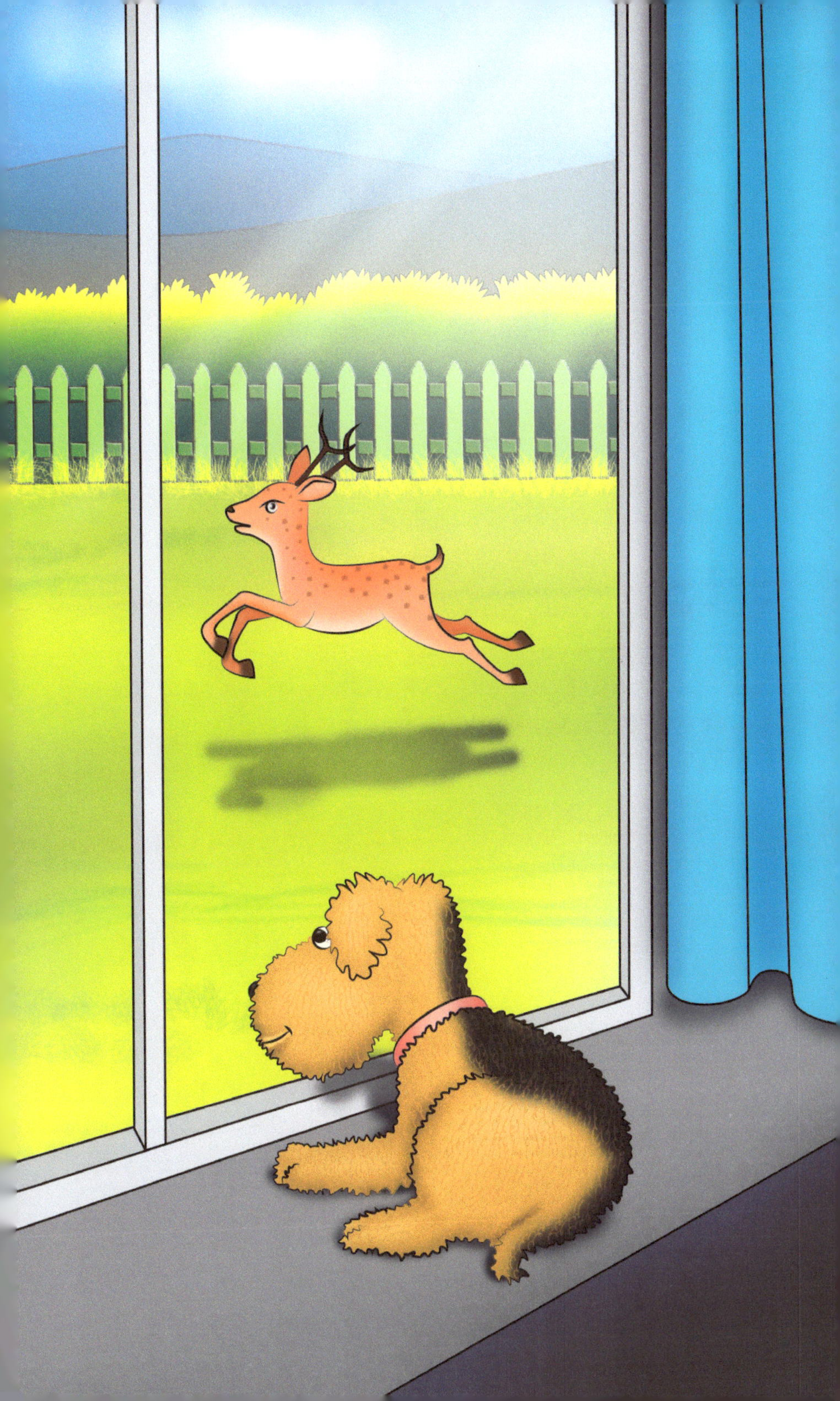

Your breed is wonderful!

See you at the Dog Park, oh, wait ... how come they don't call it a “Dog Bark”? But I digress. Ha!

**The End**

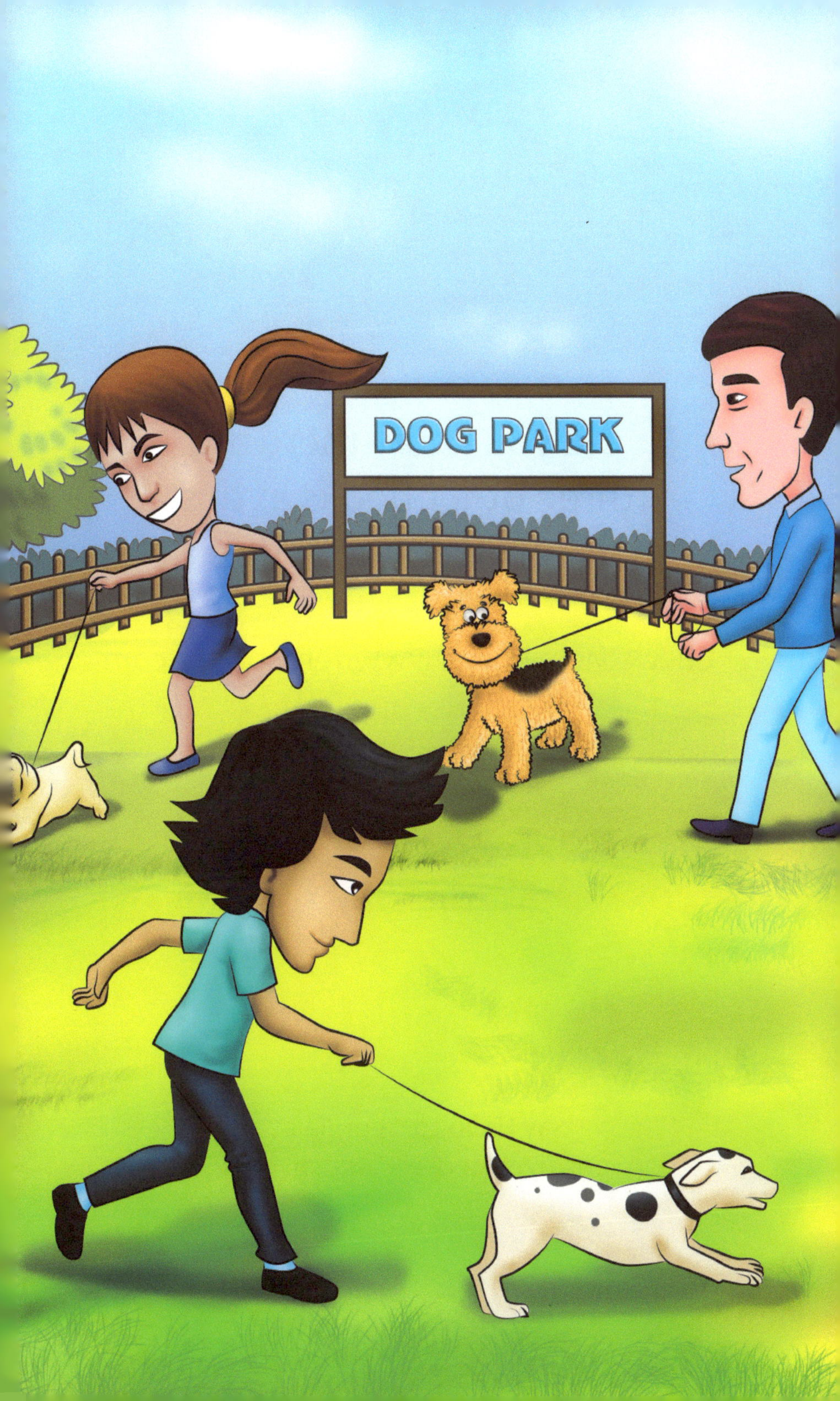
DOG PARK

Did you know there are three other books in this Juvenile fiction series?

Check them out at www.ferrisbooks.com

Say Hello to Georgia at
positivelygeorgia@gmail.com

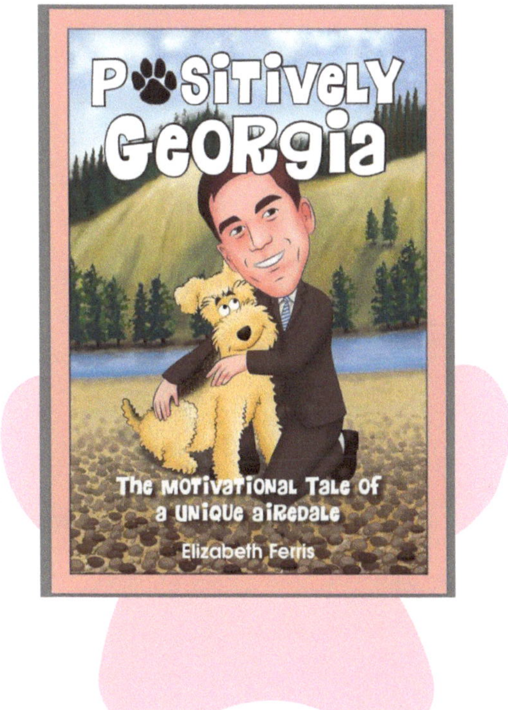


"Positively Georgia, the Motivational Tale of a Unique Airedale"

Meet Georgia, a bright-eyed and furry tailed Airedale Terrier with a very positive outlook on life.

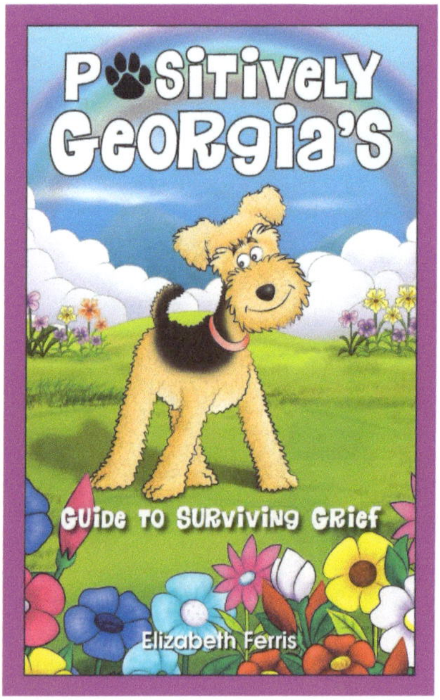


"Positively Georgia's Guide to Surviving Grief" aims to help teens and adults deal positively with the loss of a loved one.

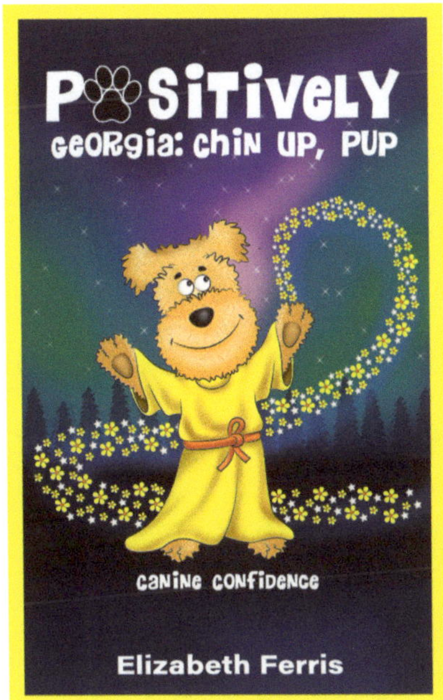


"Positively Georgia: Chin Up, Pup", aims at helping teens, young adults and adults realize their inner potential, build up their self-confidence, and follow their dreams.

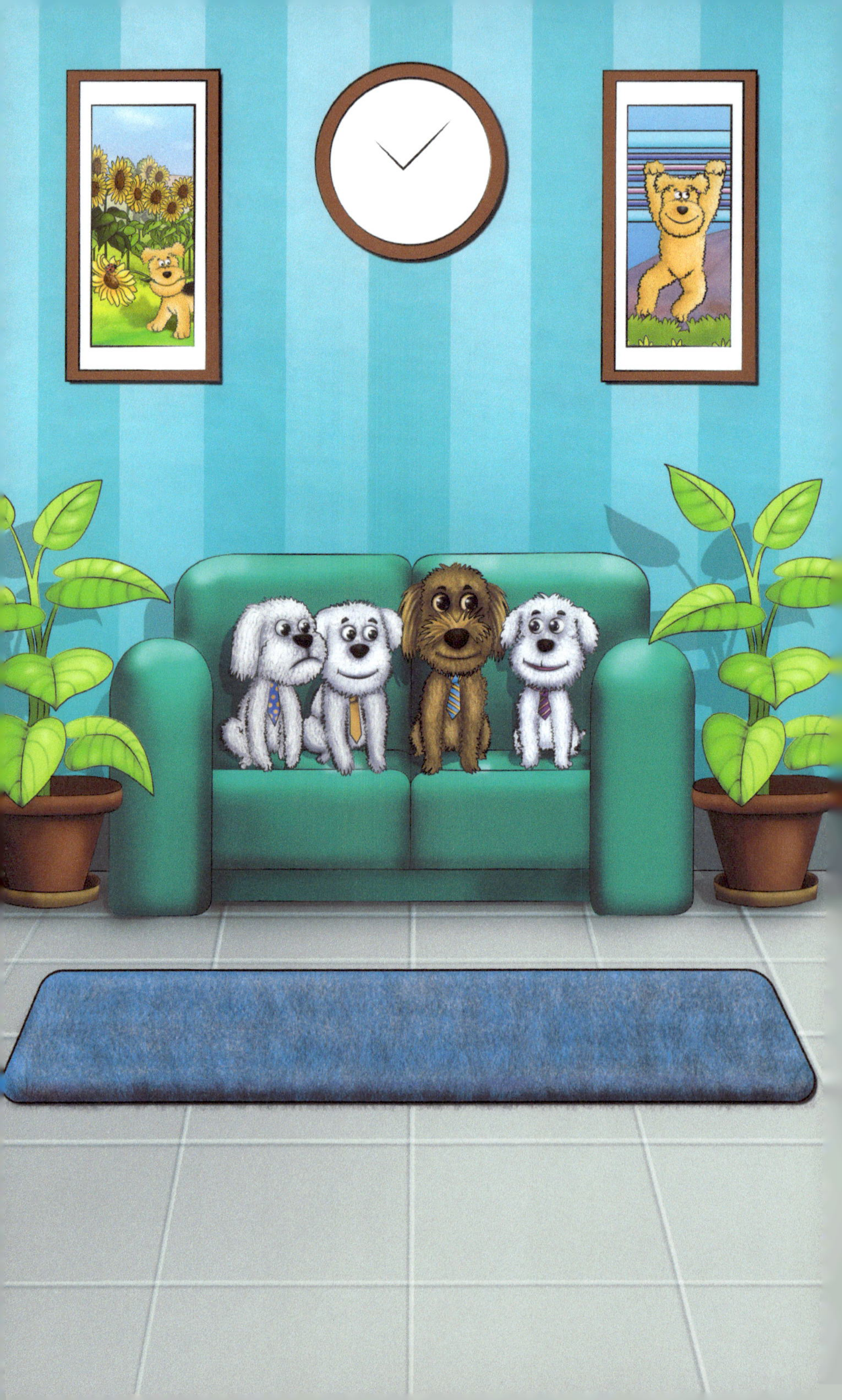

"Colorful drawings, good message for children and adults. Motivational. Story is written from the dogs point of view about interactions with other creatures. Good take away messages within, complete with the occasional poop joke."

Review by Ollie – Havanesse

"This Airedale is spreading peace, love, joy and hope one book at a time. These books are great for all breeds, shedders and non shedders alike. "

Review by Leo, Baxter and Griffin – Coton de Tulear

CPSIA information can be obtained
at www.ICGtesting.com
Printed in the USA
LVHW071034151021
700534LV00008B/568

*9781777908614*